Oil Pulling for Cleanse

The Oil Pulling Cleanse Handbook for Beginners

Table of Contents

Chapter 1 – Introduction

Chapter 2 – The Benefits

Chapter 3 – How it Works

Chapter 4 – A How to Guide

Chapter 5 – Creating a Routine

Conclusion

Introduction

Simply put, oil pulling is the process of swishing one of many different types of vegetable oil around in your mouth in order to draw the toxins out of your body through your mouth. It's a practice that's meant to cleanse the body thorough your mouth, by drawing toxins out so that you can spit them out instead of leaving them in your body. It's considered a folk remedy because not only is it a homeopathic and completely natural remedy, but because there are very few scientific research studies to provide evidence to support its benefits. However, there are plenty of those that have first-hand experience with the practice that have seen great changes after beginning their oil pulling routine. If you search the web for a few minutes, you'll find numerous first hand reports of normal, everyday people that have included oil pulling into their daily life and found great successes with it.

Oil pulling is promoted as an Ayurvedic practice. It is mentioned in the Charake Samhita, which dates back to somewhere in between 300 to 500 CE. The text called it a technique that was able to improve oral health, but it also said that it was capable of treating diseases like asthma, diabetes, and eczema. Unfortunately, there were no clearly written records of actual experiences or research done back then to prove the claims. Even now, there is a significant lack of research and evidence to back up those claims, there are a few studies that have proven that it does reduce oral plaque and gingivitis while improving the overall health and well-being of your mouth.

People claim that it is a significantly better option than normal mouthwash because there is no taste that lingers in your mouth afterwards, there is no staining caused by its use, there are no known cases of allergic reactions linked with oil pulling, and it is quickly and easily found in many households. One of the biggest arguments for that opinion is the fact that mouthwashes are all made with a variety of man-made chemicals and contain absolutely nothing that is organic or earth-made, while oil pulling is done with a simple, earth-made oil. Yes, in order to make the oil it has to be processed in a specific way, but the components are still all natural and completely organic (as long as you buy the organically made brands.)

As vegetable oils became more popular and the multitude of benefits that oil pulling can provide were uncovered and publicized, oil pulling became established as a popular alternative medicine and complementary addition to conventional medicine. While it was exposed and brought out to the public eye, it's still a very unpopular practice and it's not something that can be considered well know. It's one of those things that most people won't hear about in their lifetime, because it isn't the type of thing that many people talk about or look into. Most people don't even know that it exists, though that could change at any moment. Celebrities like Gwyneth Paltrow and Shailene Woodley have been reported to be daily practitioners of oil pulling. Just like with everything else, when a celebrity does it, it suddenly becomes much more popular. So there may be an increase in oil pulling as a legitimate form of homeopathic treatment, both for those with current oral health issues and for those that want to avoid them and boost the aesthetic appeal of their mouth and teeth.

When I first looked into it, it had nothing to do with celebrities or the hopes of hopping onto a trend before it begins. I looked into oil pulling because my gum line was receding and I wanted to find a natural way to get healthier gums. After a short amount of research, I found that there are no products sold in stores for this kind of problem, and there is no dentist-approved method to deal with it either. So I kept looking, and I found that the only guaranteed cure that a dentist can provide is a surgery. I don't have enough money to worry about an expensive dental surgery, and the idea of having someone probing into my mouth just isn't attractive to me, but I was worried about the health of my mouth. So I searched the internet until I came across oil pulling. It was the only thing aside from gargling salt water that seemed to have any merit or healing value. After a couple of hours of research, I decided that oil pulling was probably my best bet.

So I tried it. I checked my kitchen and found some olive oil. It was the only thing I had beyond regular vegetable oil, so I started with that. I read online that it was best to do it twice daily, so I got motivated and put time into it. It was difficult at first and I was highly skeptical. The texture and the feeling of the oil in my mouth was strange, and the flavor was so hard to put my finger on that I couldn't decide if it existed or not. I wanted to swallow at least once every minute, and I wanted to spit it out at least twice as many times. I only lasted ten on my first try, it was just too difficult for me to complete the task.

I gave myself a half an hour window of time to contemplate whether or not I should continue. I'd never had anything in my mouth that was quite like the oil, and I didn't have a dentist or a doctor standing there to guarantee my results. But I tried again. I got through fifteen minutes that time, and then I kept going and eventually I got better at lasting through a whole twenty minutes. I developed my own system to distract myself so that the time would go by faster and I wouldn't feel the need to swallow or spit prematurely. After a week, my teeth were both whiter and brighter. My gums were pinker. Everything looked so much healthier in my mouth, so I decided to head to the store.

I'd read that sesame oil and coconut oil were the two best options. Coconut oil is generally manufactured organically, and when I compared prices it was easy to see that sesame oil was the cheaper option. So I brought some home with me. The sesame oil tasted like an Asian sesame seed and kale salad. It's one of my favorite parts of going out for any kind of Asian food, so I was pleasantly surprised. During my first swish with it, I realized that I probably should have guessed that it would taste like that. This oil was easier, though part of that had to be due to the week of experience that I had with the olive oil. It didn't hurt that it tasted better too.

I've read testimonials from other people that said that sesame oil was too strong for them. I've read other testimonials that said that people thought that coconut oil felt like non-animal based fat sitting in their mouth. From what I gathered, if you don't enjoy sesame oil because you think that it tastes too strong, give it a few days. See if anything changes. If you can't get used to it and you still don't like it, you might want to move to olive oil. Though you should always keep in mind that the best way to get the most out of your oil pulling routine is to alternate between different oils. If you absolutely can't stand it, then you can't stand it, but if you can manage to stand a variety of these oils throughout your oil pulling routine, then you'll get the most out of it.

By the end of my first month, I was completely satisfied with the health of my gums. The recession had stopped, and I'm positive that it even healed itself at least a little bit. The inflammation at the back of my mouth where my final wisdom tooth still rests has gone down. My teeth could handle hot and cold better than before. I had a full one hundred and ten percent of skepticism resting on my shoulder that first time that I spooned a mouthful of oil in between my lips, but I'm more than happy that I tried it. The overall health of my mouth has improved greatly, and I'm proud to smile now with my full set of pearly whites showing. I have fewer headaches as well, and I feel less congested overall.

The phrase "oil pulling" as it is used today became popular in the 1990s after being used by one of the first people that ever adopted the process. His name was Lt Col Tummala Koteswara Rao and he was based in Bangalore, South India. Rao was enthusiastically active in trying to spread the word about oil pulling. He was completely convinced that it was beneficial to the entire world, and that other people needed to hear about it. Oil pulling is an ancient Ayurvedic practice, and he believed in it so wholeheartedly that he wanted other people to experience the benefits of its practice. He wrote articles about it in order to better inform the world's popular, and allowed himself to be interviewed about the benefits and the process. All of his interviews and articles were published in multiples languages at various times and delivered around the world. Still, homeopathic cures and treatments always meet with skepticism, much like my own when I first came across the practice. While Rao did his best to spread the word and inform people about the benefits of oil pulling, not everyone listened to what he had to say, which could explain why so few people know about it today.

Rao came across oil pulling by reading a paper written by Dr. F. Karach that was presented to the All Ukrainian Association of the Academy of Science of the USSR. The paper advocated the process of swishing vegetable oil as opposed to gargling it, which was the norm for most other mouth cleansing processes. It stated that Siberian shamans used sunflower oil to practice oil pulling for over a century's worth of time. Sesame seed oil is currently considered the traditional oil used for oil pulling, though recent endorsements for coconut oil have made it grow in popularity among oil pullers in the Western world.

It is said that the paper was widely distributed in 1991 in various different German magazines. The publicity was there, but the research wasn't. Not enough attention was generated by those that could research it, which is to be expected in a world filled with cancer and a variety of other so-far-uncurable diseases that need to be researched and studied. There aren't enough scientific studies to officially back up the beneficial claims of oil pulling through scientific evidence, but those that have tried it will all sing its praises. If you look online, you will find a variety of testimonies from a variety of people, all saying the same thing; oil pulling works.

Chapter Two – The Benefits

One of the first questions that you might have when it comes to adding something new into your life is simply, "Why?" Why is oil pulling something that you should introduce into your daily routine? The answer is simple and complicated at the same time; by removing toxins from your mouth, oil pulling will improve your overall health. But that's not all that you want to know, and there are plenty of details to share and go over.

There are thousands of personal stories online that rate oil pulling as "refreshing" and "incredible." Some even go as far as to call it a transforming experience. That's because the effects that they were looking for when they started oil pulling were realized. People have reported whiter teeth within just five days. Those that go into oil pulling with bleeding or sensitive gums come out of it saying that they no longer suffer from either of those things. Those that practice oil pulling regularly have said that their dentists are impressed, and can find little to no plaque on their teeth.

Just like with every other new thing to catch the eye of a group of people, there are critics that like to say that these positive benefits work the same way that a placebo or sugar pill does, but the facts speak against that. There isn't very much research done on the topic of oil pulling, but every study and experiment that has been done to test it has proven that it has positive benefits. Not every claim has been proven, but a good majority of them have been.

Simply put, oil pulling will improve your overall oral health. The fact that you're removing toxins from your mouth probably already made that point obvious, but there are key details that you might not have guessed. Oil pulling will strengthen your teeth, gums, and jaw. It can lower the risk of infections and lower the count of bacteria by removing it from your mouth. Imagine you've just had oral surgery, or you have a concern like gingivitis or receding gums. Oil pulling will draw toxins away and improve your oral health by removing the causes of most oral health problems.

A study was done in 2008 to test the effects of oil pulling on a group of people that had been infected with Streptococcus mutans. There were ten people involved in the study in total; ten were put into a control group that were left to live their life as they normally would and the other ten was introduced to oil pulling. Plaque and saliva samples were taken from all of the people that were involved in the study during the entire duration. The group that was tasked with testing out oil pulling were given sesame oil and the control group was given a chlorhexidine mouthwash solution. Both groups were told to swish for ten minutes every morning before brushing their teeth. The researchers that oversaw this study took samples from the people in both groups at twenty-four hours, forty-eight hours, one week, and then the final time two weeks after the study began. The saliva samples proved that there was a dramatic decrease in Streptococcus mutans in the group that used oil pulling every morning. The result was clear; oil pulling is an effective addition to a normal oral cleansing routine and can help prevent and improve oral health.

There are also claims of oil pulling improving the health beyond just your mouth. It's reported to soothe headaches and lower the amount of times a week that they reoccur. There's a man that also claims to have cured his arthritis through the simple practice of oil pulling. It's known to support normal kidney function. Others say that it will clear your sinuses and prevent bad breath. The claims go as far as to say that it can protect against heart disease and Alzheimer's disease as well.

It's not just good when it comes to healing bodily ailments, it's a good preventative as well. The simplest form of that is found in the way that the oil clings to the surfaces in your mouth. The remnants of oil act as a barrier against germs and bacteria, stopping them from sticking around. Considering the amount of things that come in contact with your mouth, you can imagine how useful that would be. Beyond that, the consistent action of pulling the bacteria and germs out of your mouth on a daily basis leaves you with a cleaner mouth. That prevents tooth decay, cavities, gingivitis, and all kinds of other bacteria-born oral troubles.

But it doesn't stop at the health improvements; oil pulling can whiten and brighten your teeth too. It only takes about a week to see an obvious visual improvement, and it's certainly much less expensive and time consuming than any of the chemically based at-home whitening treatments that you can find in the toothpaste aisle or at your local dentist. It is also said that oil pulling reduces acne. It makes sense that a process that is designed to draw toxins out of your body would be able to lower the amount of little red bumps caused by clogged pores. If you add the benefits of whitening your teeth and reducing acne, it's easy to see that oil pulling can also improve your self-esteem and how you see yourself by improving your appearance. Those are two of some of the biggest appearance related concerns, especially when it comes to teens and young adults. If the solution is as simple as swishing some oil around your mouth for a few minutes a day, why not try it?

What is arguably the best thing about oil pulling is the fact that you don't need anything expensive or chemically enhanced to practice it. Oil pulling is a completely natural, homeopathic remedy that has absolutely zero lasting negative side effects. There are no harsh chemicals involved, just the simple action of swishing oil around your mouth for a little while. That was what drew me to it originally, especially considering the fact that the only other option for oral improvement for me was an expensive surgery. There are no harsh chemicals in these vegetable oils, especially if you're buying organically. So there is relief for those that are conscious about those kinds of things. And the oils themselves are inexpensive. I paid about four dollars for my first bottle of sesame oil, and the general price of the cheaper line of organic coconut oil is somewhere around ten dollars.

Chapter Three – How It Works

While there aren't very many scientific studies that have been completely on the subject of oil pulling, it is known that the oil draws out toxins as you swish it around your mouth. It also holds them in, so that you're not drawing them out just to stick them to another part of your mouth. Pulling out the toxins cleans your mouth, which enhances your oral health as a whole.

It is said that you can estimate a person's general and overall health just by looking into their mouth. If you think about it in normal, everyday terms, it makes sense. Your mouth is a breeding ground for over six hundred different types of bacteria, fungi, yeast, and a variety of other microorganisms that like to live inside the steamy, dark, slimy, and warm little hiding spots in your mouth. It's even said that you can find more bacteria in one mouth than there are people on the planet. Humans swallow saliva when they eat, drink, and even just at regular points throughout the day. That means that all of those things that are hiding out in your mouth are very likely to be found in your stomach as well. Your stomach directs its contents to the rest of your body through digestion. It is a well-known fact that any bacteria or infectious material that is found in your mouth can make its way throughout your blood stream. With that being said, it's obvious that your mouth would be one of the first places to think about improving on if you want to raise your overall health.

When you spit out the oil, the toxins leave your body with it. That simple fact cleans your mouth better than brushing your teeth or swishing with mouthwash, and it's natural so there are no chemicals involved. There is no evidence that can prove how oil pulling works the way that it does, but it isn't difficult to believe the claims of its benefits once you've seen how well it works.

There is no proof to define just how far oil pulling goes to draw out toxins. Some would believe that it only serves its purpose inside of your mouth, while others believe that it can pull toxins out of your entire body. There are claims and reports of oil pulling curing arthritis and ailing headaches. Some people even believe that it cures acne and other skin conditions.

The next way that the process works comes after the oil has been spit out. Miniscule residue from the oil coats your mouth and acts as a protective barrier against bacteria. It's like a shield that stops germs from clinging to the inside of your mouth, which helps keep it clean long after the oil has been spit out.

Overall, it is said that oil pulling will strengthen your gums, teeth, and jaw. It's known to prevent gingivitis and rumored to prevent cavities as well. Drawing all of the toxins out of your mouth will save your stomach the hassle of dealing with them, which will boost your immune system by allowing it to deal with other threats instead. It has an overall detoxifying affect, and efficiently cleans out your body.

The side effects of all of the good things that oil pulling can do for you include better sleep that will bring on an increase in energy. Oil pulling helps reduce the severity of headaches and the amount of times that you have them too, which could also be a factor in the cause of the increase in energy. It's also known that oil pulling clears out your sinuses, which could improve your visits to the ear, nose, and throat doctor. It's been reported to have helped with cases of aches and pains too, which could be as big as aiding in arthritis relief. After all of the oral health improvements that oil pulling can provide, it's obvious that it will also improve your breath and cure bad breath completely by getting rid of the source.

Some people use oil pulling as a hangover cure. Other people use it because it helps to get rid of skin problems, like eczema, acne, and psoriasis. It decreases the amount of breakouts for those that suffer from acne. If eczema is an issue for you, it helps to heal your existing problem areas and reduces the itching completely. It's also known to balance out your hormones.

There are only two things that can be considered negative parts of the oil pulling process, and they aren't even all that negative. The first, and most obvious, is the fact that it takes twenty minutes of time to take full advantage of the process. It's easy to feel like you've avoided wasting time by doing other things while you participate in the oil pulling process. There are many people that like to read while they pull their oil. Others prepare their breakfast, or do some other productive part of their morning routine while their mouth is busy with oil pulling. The only part of your body that will be unable to be used for other things is your mouth, so the potential amount of things that you can do with the twenty minutes that you spend pulling oil is endless.

The other negative side effect is that for some people, there will be a bit of tooth sensitivity involved for the first few days. This isn't felt by most people, but if you do feel it, just continue. Be kind to your teeth and avoid anything that it overly hot or overly cold. It should only take a few days for your teeth to get used to the oil pulling process, and then you will never feel that sensitivity because of oil pulling ever again.

With all of the positive benefits that can come from oil pulling, and so few reasons not to do it, it might be time to start considering it more seriously; especially if you already have a preexisting oral health problem that you would like to address.

Chapter Four – A Simple How-To

Now that you've decided to implement oil pulling as a part of your daily life, you need to come up with a routine in order to ensure that you reap the benefits in the most complete and efficient way. The first thing to do is to decide what type of oil you'd like to use. Sesame oil is the most often critically acclaimed "perfect oil" for oil pulling. Coconut oil is a newer discovery, but the media has advertised it enough that it's beginning to rise in the ranks. Sunflower oil is credited as the first known type of oil to be used for oil pulling. The most efficient way to make sure that you get the most out of oil pulling is to alternate oils. Each different type of oil is acclaimed for different reasons, so it stands to reason that using all of them would give you the best end result.

In order to be the most effective, oil pulling is performed by placing approximately a tablespoon of chilled organic oil into the mouth before swishing it around for about ten to twenty minutes before spitting it out. Some people choose to go for a full twenty minutes. It's argued that twenty minutes is the perfect amount of time to soak up the toxins in your mouth without risking them being reabsorbed by your body. You don't want to do it for too long though, because it is thought that doing so might allow the toxins to sink back into your body. The oil mixes with your saliva, turning it into a white liquid. As the oil is continuously swished around your mouth, it absorbs toxins and more often than not, ends up turning thick and white. When the oil has reached this desired state, it is spit out before the bacteria and toxins have the chance to be reabsorbed by the mouth, teeth, gums and tongue.

It's important to remember to start the oil pulling sometime right after you first wake up in the morning. You don't want to eat or brush your teeth first, for more than one reason. Most people aren't too fond of having oil in their mouth, so it's easier to successfully get through the process without feeling a little sick to your stomach if it's empty. An empty stomach will also increase the production of your salivary glands, which improves the efficiency of the process.

Step One: Measure out a small spoonful of oil and then swish it around your mouth. The exact amount isn't that important, but it should be enough to move around your mouth while not being so much that you feel as though you've really got a mouth full. The goal is to continue to do it for ten to twenty minutes before you spit it out. The recommended time varies, depending on where you look or who you ask. There isn't a noted "perfect amount of time" to swish the oil for, but there are many that say that twenty minutes is the perfect amount of time. They argue that it gives the oil enough time to draw out and absorb toxins without giving those toxins enough time to sink back into your mouth. It's not always easy, and the first few times are definitely a little difficult, so keep that in mind. There are some people that have a really hard time trying to keep the oil in their mouth. It's not the kind of thing that anyone normally has in their mouth on a regular basis, so it's going to take a little time to get used to it. If you find that it's more unpleasant than you're willing to deal with, try it again a few times, just to see if it gets easier. If it doesn't, then use a different oil. Just remember that oil pulling is the most effective when you are capable of alternating between different oils. Each different oil has different qualities and brings different benefits.

Don't swallow it, no matter what, especially after you've been going for a few minutes. The oil soaks up toxins, and while your body is equipped to take care of safely processing them, the purpose of this is to get the toxins out of your body, not to put them in deeper. It helps if you keep your chin tucked down a little bit, so the oil steers clear of the back of your mouth. It lowers the chances of the muscles in the back of your mouth tensing and trying to force you to swallow through triggering the physical movements that lead up to it.

If you ever feel like you're going to swallow the oil and you can't help yourself, spit it out. It's as simple as that. If it hasn't been that long, you can always just start over with a new spoonful of oil. Swallowing the oil is generally harmless, but you have to remember that the point of this practice is to fill it with toxins and expel them from your body. The last thing that you want to do is swallow the oil so that the toxins go deeper into your body than they were originally. There are no lasting health defects that are earned by swallowing the oil, but it can irritate your stomach. The most severe side effect of swallowing your oil is diarrhea. Still, even if you don't end up with a negative side effect, you don't want to swallow the oil.

I get through the time by pressing the tip of my tongue up against the bottom of my front teeth so that I can push the oil through the spaces in between my teeth. After I've done that for a little while, I rotate the direction that I push the oil and try to push it through the rest of my teeth. It's more difficult than I thought that it would be, and usually by the time I've managed to push the oil in between all of my teeth a couple dozen times, the time is up. I think it's the fact that I turn it into a game that makes it easier to get through the time, because it takes my mind off of it. I stop thinking about the feel of the oil in my mouth, and I also stop thinking about waiting for the minutes to tick by. I set a timer on my cell phone to make sure that I don't end up going on for too long.

So if you don't like my approach, I suggest finding another method. You could sit in front of your computer and check up on things, read a book, or paint your nails. There are a few people that said that they chose to do it in the shower, that way they could focus on cleaning their bodies while they were cleaning their mouth. It made it easier, because they focused less on what was going on in their mouth and more on what they needed to do in order to complete their showers. Simply put; anything that helps you keep swishing the oil around your mouth without swallowing it is a good idea. Just don't let time run away with you. If you think you're going to have trouble remembering when to spit the oil out, set an alarm.

One thing that can trigger the desire to swallow is a full mouth. If you feel as though your mouth has become too full at any point, you can always spit a little bit out. It's happened to me a few times, and I wasn't sure whether it would hinder the process. It doesn't. Just don't spit out too much and continue on as though you never stopped.

Step Two: When it is time to spit out your oil, remember to spit it out in a trash can. Don't spit it out in the sink, especially if you have a septic system. The toxins and the oil might clog up your pipes, and nobody wants that.

Step Three: Once you've spit the oil out into the trash, you can rinse your mouth with warm water. The heat in the water cleans better than cold water, and it gets any of the remaining oil out of your mouth. It's best to completely clear out your mouth before you move on, that way you mouth is at its cleanest.

Step Four: Once you've rinsed thoroughly, you can brush your teeth like normal. Make sure that you brush completely, and don't skip out on the time you spend on it. Oil pulling is a wonderful method to add to your normal oral health routine, but it isn't meant to completely replace all other steps in the process. Feel free to use mouthwash when you're done.

It has been noted that some people experience something that is very similar to a detox when they first begin oil pulling. It's rare, but it does happen. The process of drawing toxins out of the body also brings more to the surface, which can cause symptoms that are cold or flu-like. Some of these symptoms can include headache, mild congestion, mucus drainage, and other similar side effects. Fortunately, all of these symptoms are temporary, and none of them should last much longer than a week at the most. Continue on as normal and they will clear up on their own. Consider it your body's way of creating a physical manifestation to show you what it's getting rid of.

Chapter Five – Creating A Routine

It's not always easy to add new things to your daily routine. If you find that you're having trouble remembering to set aside the time for oil pulling, then you might want to find a more obvious way to push it into your life. Just like when you try to add anything else to your daily routine, you need to find a way to remind yourself. For the first week, I kept my sesame oil on my nightstand, right next to my bed. That way, I could wake up, rub my eyes, sit up, and pour myself a cap full. I measured it, and it was just about the same amount as a spoonful. Then I could sit in bed and literally start my day off with oil pulling. After that week, I put the sesame oil back into the kitchen and managed to make my way in to grab it within a half an hour of waking up every morning.

Most people brush their teeth first thing in the morning, so if leaving your pulling oil beside your bed doesn't sound like a good idea to you, it might be better to leave it in the bathroom beside your toothbrush. Then whenever you go to reach for it first thing in the morning, you can remind yourself that the oil comes first.

Other people remind themselves with notes and alarms, setting visual or audio reminders to shock the addition to their schedule into their lives. It's more difficult to forget something that you see every day. That was the concept behind leaving the sesame oil beside my bed. Leave a note for yourself on your bathroom mirror, so that you see it a few times a day. If you have a phone that you use as your alarm, you can even set a note on that to remind you about your oil pulling.

Beyond just remembering to do it, you need to decide how you're going to schedule it. Are you going to try oil pulling once a day? Twice a day? Are you going to use sesame oil? What about coconut? Or sunflower oil? When I started doing it, I read somewhere that it was good to do it once as soon as you wake up, and then once again before bed. (As long your stomach is empty at the time, it will work to its highest potential.) I only had olive oil, so I only used olive oil. When I realized that it was working, I immediately went out to the store and bought myself some sesame oil, just to make sure that I got the best results possible. I was hesitant about continuing with the olive oil because I didn't see it on anyone's recommended lists anywhere.

The best way to get the most out of oil pulling is to alternate between oils. Sesame and coconut are the two top contenders, though sunflower oil is credited as the first oil to be used for oil pulling. There are some people that prefer one over the other for both sides. All three oils have been proven more than capable of removing plaque and simple, everyday bacteria that might be found inside of your mouth. Alternate days, so that you can get the benefits of all three. You might also want to try experimenting with different brands of oils to find which one you like best. Some people find it's easier with thicker oils, others enjoy the more watered down versions. The texture of the oil in your mouth is going to greatly affect whether or not you want to spit it out immediately or not. It'll make the experience easier, and easier is always better.

If you're going to use coconut oil, be sure to read the labels on the container thoroughly. The media has raised the awareness of coconut oil and it's rising in popularity, but some coconut oil comes with a high MCT (medium chain triglyceride) level. MCT is known to cause symptoms that mimic that of a hangover in some people when they're exposed to it frequently. One way to avoid that, beyond reading the label thoroughly or researching the product that you want to use before you buy it, is to make sure that you get unrefined, organic coconut oil. There are extra additives in refined coconut oil, and the process that it goes through takes away some of its natural components. Basically, it's like diluting the product and adding things into it that you don't want.

Everyone likes being able to use the things that they buy for more than one purpose, so if you do decide to use coconut oil, there are other things that you can use it for as well. It's a great hair care product, especially when it comes to healing split or dry ends. Just remember that it isn't always easy to get out of your hair, so you don't want to use more than three tablespoons at a time. All you have to do is heat it in the microwave for about a minute or so and then spread it into your hair like you would if you were dying your hair with it. Keep it away from your scalp, because your scalp already has enough natural oils in it that it doesn't need that help. Then leave it in for a couple of hours and wash it out.

In 2010, an article about a study on oil pulling was accepted into the Asia Journal of Public Health. The study researched the effects of oil pulling when it comes to microorganisms in different biofilm models. They tested corn oil, rice bran oil, coconut oil, sesame oil, palm oil, sunflower oil, and soy bean oil. They were tested against the Streptococcus mutas KPSK2, Candida albicans ATCC 13803, and Lactobacillus casei ATCC 6363. The experiments were conducted on microtiter plates that were coated in saliva to mimic the environment that you would find in a mouth. In every experiment you need controls to make sure that the evidence that you find can be used to prove that the product that you're using is what made the change, nothing else. This experiment used saline solution and a 0.2% chlorhexiden gluconate solution (in layman's terms, it's basically normal mouthwash) as negative and positive controls. In the end, coconut oil was proven to provide antimicrobial qualities when it came in contact with the S. mutans and C. albicans. The sesame oil proved to have antibacterial qualities when it was pitted against the S. mutans. Sunflower oil was proven to host antifungal qualities when faced with C. albicans. The L. casei refused to be affected by any of the three.

This study proved a few different things. First, it gave scientific evidence and proved that oil pulling can be a successful and efficient home remedy homeopathic treatment against oral health issues. It mentioned that this success might be particularly useful in countries that are still developing, and therefore have yet to completely accomplish health care opportunities for every citizen. It also shows that coconut oil might be considered an antimicrobial, sesame oil might be considered an antibacterial, and sunflower oil might be considered an antifungal. The fact that all three oils were proven to cure and treat different things backs up the idea that you should use and alternative between all three different kinds of oil in order to get the best results from your oil pulling routine.

Avoid canola oil, cottonseed oil, corn oil, and soy oil. These oils will not produce the same benefits and results as the approved oils will. Stay away from any oils that go bad quickly, like flax oil, for obvious reasons. If your oil isn't going to stay useful for very long, you might as well not even bother with it. The last thing that you want is to put a spoonful of it into your mouth and realize that it's gone bad.

Once you've decided on which types of oil to use, you have to figure out how often you want to do it. Most people stick to a simple once a day routine, where they practice oil pulling right after they wake up and then go about their day as normal. Other people, like myself, choose to do it twice a day; once in the morning before doing anything else and then once at night right before going to bed. It's also been said be Dr. Bruce Fife that you can boost your efforts by practicing oil pulling before every meal. That's generally only advice that's given to people with more severe dental or oral health issues, but it is a viable option for anyone.

The bottom line is, oil pulling is a highly beneficial practice that can be added to your daily routine. For the low cost of twenty to forty minutes of your time (depending on how often you decide to do it) you can greatly improve your oral health, and through that improve the rest of your body as well. If you're not sure whether or not oil pulling will benefit you the way that you want it to, just try it. You can give yourself a week-long trial period to give yourself a chance to see what adding oil pulling into your daily routine will do for you. You won't lose anything by giving yourself the opportunity to see improvement.